"We aren't telling going to be easy; we are telling you it's going to be worth it"

Welcome

Welcome to The Sober Experiment® by Bee Sober. Our aim, through Sober Experiment® and Bee Sober is, not only to change your relationship with alcohol for good, but to also support, inspire and motivate you to achieve a successful and sustained sobriety through our community.

We sometimes don't realize how often we drink alcohol, or, how much we depend on that nightly glass of wine or beer. While drinking in moderation isn't all bad, taking one month off will positively impact your future drinking choices. With just 30 days off, a whole new world could open up for you. The 30-day mark is only the beginning — but already a number of positive changes will become very apparent. You could find yourself losing a few extra pounds, you will feel happier, have more energy, brighter skin and get a better night's sleep.

This member's pack belongs to

....

The Sober Experiment® by Bee Sober
Copyright 2020.

All rights reserved. No portion of this book may be reproduced in any form without permission from the publisher. The opinions expressed in this book are those held by the authors and should not be taken as advice. This journal is not intended to replace the advice of your doctor or medical professional, if you have a physical dependence on alcohol. Our programme is intended for those who have emotional dependency on alcohol and wish to cut down or quit drinking alcohol for good. If at any point you feel unwell during your experiment, please seek medical and professional advice immediately.

Authors: Bee Sober

When you reach 30 days sober, you will notice a definite improvement in your mood, with a more positive outlook on life and a renewed sense of purpose.

Studies have also shown that giving up for just one month could have positive long-term health benefits by reducing the number of drinking days later in the year.

We would like to take this opportunity to thank you for choosing Bee Sober to support you through your sober journey. May we wish you all the luck and love in the world.

YOU'VE GOT THIS!

Sober Survival Tips

- Make sobriety your number one priority for a while. You WILL make it.

- Reward progress. It's important that you acknowledge the fact that making changes to your lifestyle can be difficult and that you reward yourself if you are making progress.

- Take it one day at a time. Thinking about quitting for a long time can seem daunting. Taking things one day at a time is more achievable.

- Avoid temptation. In the early stages, it's a good idea to avoid situations where you may be tempted to drink. This could mean opting out of the weekly pub quiz for a while, or if you tend to drink when eating out, try going to restaurants that don't sell alcohol or simply volunteer to drive.

- Keep hydrated.

- Commit fully. Sobriety isn't something you can achieve with minimal effort.

- Keep it simple, eat well (especially before your drinking hour), and make a plan that lists your triggers and how bad drinking is for you (relationships, as a parent, financially, living life to the full, workwise etc.).

- Stay positive. Quitting is more difficult if you have a negative attitude.

- Use the Facebook support group. Almost everyone who struggles to quit drinking requires some form of peer support. As with any goal, quitting alcohol is easier if you have friends supporting you. The group can encourage you to stay sober and help you find other healthy ways to have fun.

- Read self-help books - These can boost your confidence and motivate you to stay sober.

- Write down what it is you want. How do you want to live? Now FOCUS on those things.

- Have faith. When you believe sobriety is possible, you're more likely to achieve it.

- Avoid shops after 1-2pm, for as long as it takes (this is an amazing strategy to stop 'absent-minded' buying of booze).

- Try to think about today only. Focus on getting through this minute, this hour, this day.

- If you have a family to feed and cooking in the evening is a trigger, do as much preparation as you can on the weekend and let yourself indulge in as many take-outs as you might need to on crazy days. Leave the chores if you need to keep calm.

- Think of your first 30 days as an at-home rehab and treat yourself to the help you need to keep the evening stress at a minimum.

- Open a book, open a browser, open your mind. The keys are out there.

- You don't HAVE to drink.

- If you are still really struggling, please ask for help. Getting sober is hard to do on your own.

You can do this!!!

What can you expect during the first 30 days?

The First 24 Hours

Very shortly after your last drink, your liver has a huge task to undertake. It must detoxify your bloodstream to prevent alcohol poisoning. As the alcohol is processed, it changes the alcohol into acetaldehyde, a highly poisonous substance and a known carcinogen. This toxin, although only in the body for a very short time before being converted to acetate, has the potential to cause significant and irreversible damage. The typical hangover symptoms, or tremors and nausea, are a direct result of the presence of acetaldehyde.

Due to the sudden and dramatic rise in sugar levels (from whatever you drank), insulin is also produced by your pancreas to remove the sugar from your bloodstream. This causes a temporary imbalance whilst your body tries to stabilise the blood sugars and causes you to crave carbohydrate. A fantastic explanation for why you crave a stodgy meal (junk food) after drinking. The best way to deal with this is to drink plenty of water and eat healthy wholesome foods to rebalance.

Days 2-3

Blood sugar levels settle, and the hangover is all but gone. However, you may still feel sleepy, grumpy and unwell overall. In heavier drinkers, withdrawal symptoms can include sweating, increased heart rate, tremors, anxiety and adverse mood. This can be a dangerous stage for heavy drinkers, and you may need medical support. By day three, you should be feeling 'back to normal' but your body has only just started its amazing journey to sobriety.

End of Week One

You might feel a little bored. This is good. It means your creative brain is switching on. Alcohol has numbed this. It is at this point that you can crave alcohol because you are looking for something to fill the time. You need to find new and stimulating activities to engage or re-engage in. Your body should now be rehydrated which means that you will have more energy in the day. You might have noticed a few headaches this week, but they should be subsiding as you become more hydrated. During the night, you may be feeling a bit restless. Sleep has been interrupted during your alcohol use and your body has been used to having alcohol in there to help you to fall asleep. By the end of week one and into week two, your brain starts to make the shift back to regulating its natural sleep patterns, you may feel drowsy early in the evening but be restless during the night. You have been used to having irregular sleep patterns and poor-quality sleep and your brain now has to re-learn to find chemical balance without alcohol. You should find sleep improves within the next week.

End of Week Two

Your skin, having been hydrated, starts to look healthier. You have more or less fully detoxed by this stage so sleep should have returned to normal and any anxiety you have experienced should have subsided. You have probably reduced your overall calorie intake by 2100 per week (on average) so you may notice your clothes feel more comfortable. Not everyone loses weight yet, as sometimes we crave sugar. This is due to no longer imbibing sugary alcoholic drinks, so you feel the need to substitute the sugar intake in other ways. Try to choose natural sugars where possible.

End of Week Three

After three weeks, your blood pressure starts to reduce. There is a reduced risk of stroke and heart attack and your kidneys become much healthier. Take a look at your eyes, the whites look whiter! By now, you have saved a whopping £60. Perhaps you can sign up to a local gym or invest in that hobby you wanted to take up but never did.

30 Days

Your liver is healing and already, the fat that was building up around it is reducing. Your skin is glowing, you are sleeping better, and anxiety levels are stabilised. Even if you return to drinking at this stage, you are much more likely to reduce the amount you drink for the next 6-12 months. As your liver is working better, you may find you feel well! You are now less likely to get sick as your immune system is returning to full health. The average drinker has now saved £80-£100. What will you do with this extra cash?

Make Bee-ing Sober Work for You

There is something really special about connecting like-minded people on their sobriety journey, supporting each other, cheering each other on and sharing motivational ideas.

We understand how challenging it can be to push yourself out of your comfort zone and join a group. Simply making this decision is amazing and you are demonstrating true commitment to your sobriety and your self-development.

You have done the right thing; we are proud of you and this is only the very beginning. Your exciting sober journey is about to become amazing.

We are all in this together. The key to success is in support and connection. Join our Facebook group and Sober Support Lounges, every single week, no matter how you are feeling; what cravings and self-doubt you may be experiencing - we will all be here to cheer you on.

"We care about everyone and whatever your story we can support you. Realising you are not alone can help you to be kinder to yourself".

Trust in our Tools

If you complete the activities in this member's pack, whilst carrying out The Sober Experiment®, we guarantee you will get sober. The tools in this member's pack have been developed out of a deep understanding of the psychology of addiction, to help you understand your feelings – Bee Kind to yourself!

We know along your journey, you will have both ups and downs, good days and bad days, successes and challenges. These groups are about the downs as much as the ups and actually matter even more at times when perhaps you don't feel like joining.

These are the days when your cravings might catch you off guard. We are all human and soon to be your friendly support network. Everyone here is walking in your shoes and we can all help each other to make a success plan for when the next challenging times hit.

Our mistakes can also be our major learning points.

The support from the Bee Sober team and your fellow members will leave you feeling like you floated out of our meetings on a pink fluffy cloud, able to conquer the world!

Some days you will need the group but most days the group will need you!

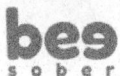

Day Counter

We have included a 30-day counter for you to count down the days of your experiment to meet your goal, one day at a time.

Daily Journal

Use the personal journal for your own recordings to track and monitor your feelings on a daily basis. Research has shown that if you write down your feelings, you process them before acting on impulse. This can be an effective way to keep you on track.

Daily Activities

The activities are intended as a tool to allow you to reflect on your sober journey. These are what worked for us and you may decide that not all of them are for you. Please use this to help yourself and remain open-minded.

Please note that you do not have to complete the activities in the format we have suggested. Some people prefer to draw pictures, record short videos or audio notes instead. This is your tool and for you to use in a way that best suits you.

30-Day Counter

Use this 30-day tracker to track your progress by crossing off the days as they pass.
Remember you have ONLY committed to a 30-day experiment – you can do this. If the worst happens, however, record what drink(s) you had, dust yourself off and get straight back on it!

1	2	3	4	5
6	7	8	9	10
11	12	13	14	15
16	17	18	19	20
21	22	23	24	25
26	27	28	29	30

"Day one or one day, you decide"

Day 1

How do I feel today? Circle the face that best represents how you feel.

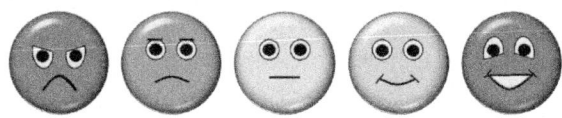

Record any observations and feelings you are experiencing, both positive and negative, in the space below.

Day 1

Day 1 - The voice in your head

The pros to drinking alcohol and the pros to not drinking alcohol. OK, let's be real. If you didn't think there would be any pros to drinking then you would never do it and if you didn't think there would be any pros to not drinking then you wouldn't be here either. We want you to be really honest with yourself here and list everything you think is good about drinking and everything you think will be good about not drinking. There is method in this madness – we promise. It'll give you a really good idea of where you are and the reason you choose to drink.

Day 1 Activity

What are your current pros of drinking alcohol and not drinking alcohol? List them here to re-visit on day 30.

Pros of drinking alcohol	Pros of not drinking alcohol

"I am not a product of my circumstances; I am a product of my decisions"

Day 2

How do I feel today? Circle the face that best represents how you feel.

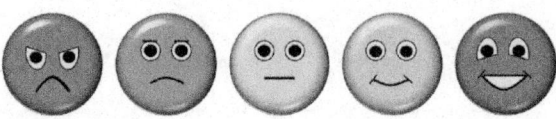

Record any observations and feelings you are experiencing, both positive and negative, in the space below.

Day 2

Day 2 - Expect the unexpected

Expect the unexpected! In the first few days and weeks of stopping drinking, it seems to be all you can think about! Ever bought a red car and suddenly all you see is red cars? Day two is about identifying the times you would normally reach for a drink and formulating an action plan for what you will do when the 'wine witch' comes calling! Preparation is key so you don't get caught off guard. These don't have to be huge activities, simply walking into another room to pour yourself a non-alcoholic drink can be enough to stop a craving in its tracks. Today is also a good day for a selfie – send it to us if you are brave!

Day 2 Activity

What is your wine or beer o'clock action plan? Write down what you will do when the voice in your head starts telling you to drink alcohol.
Take a selfie and either keep it until we prompt you to take the next one or send it to us if you're brave enough.

My Action Plan

"You must unlearn what you have learned"

Day 3

How do I feel today? Circle the face that best represents how you feel.

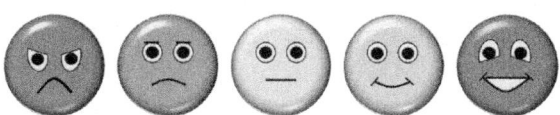

Record any observations and feelings you are experiencing, both positive and negative, in the space below.

Day 3

Day 3 - Sobriety and sleeping

Sobriety and sleep. How amazing is a good night's sleep? When was the last time you had a truly rested sleep, unbroken and long. After sleep we always feel better and sleep is proven to impact your physical and mental health. At some point within the next week (it may already have happened), you are going to experience your best night's sleep in ages. This is because alcohol impacts sleep. Ever just been tired after a night out. That is actually a hangover from the alcohol messing with your sleep! Get ready for the sleep of your life and let us know when it happens.

Day 3 Activity

When was the last time you had a decent night's sleep? How did you feel afterwards?

On what day (after stopping alcohol) did you experience your first good night's sleep? How did you feel afterwards?

"When life gets tough, remember you are tougher!"

Day 4

How do I feel today? Circle the face that best represents how you feel.

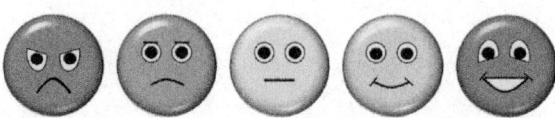

Record any observations and feelings you are experiencing, both positive and negative, in the space below.

Day 4

Day 4 - Alcohol is bad

How Alcohol is sold to you! Birthday cards, TV shows, sexy models having a beer, and "funny" signs like "one prosecco, two prosecco, three prosecco, floor" to hang in the kitchen are just some of the ways the alcohol industry sucks you in. Look around and take notice of all the ways you are drawn in and all the ways alcohol is normalised. Did you know that alcohol is an anaesthetic and used to be used in surgery until it was finally banned in the 1970s for being too toxic? Hmmmmm – strange!

Day 4 Activity

Notice all the ways alcohol is 'sold' to you. Write them down below and add to it throughout the experiment.

All the ways alcohol is 'sold' to me (advertising)

"You have no idea what you're really capable of until you get sober"

Day 5

How do I feel today? Circle the face that best represents how you feel.

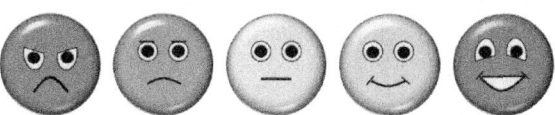

Record any observations and feelings you are experiencing, both positive and negative, in the space below.

Day 5

Day 5 - Cravings

Cravings. We crave alcohol at the strangest times. When the kids go to bed, when someone dies, when someone is born, when we are happy/sad/stressed/excited – the list goes on. What are the main reasons you use alcohol? How does alcohol help or contribute in this situation? Without alcohol, what other things can you do to ease the situation? Today it is about finding alternatives and more healthy ones at that!

Day 5 Activity

Write down the main reason(s) you use alcohol?

How will the alcohol help you in this situation?

If the alcohol will not help, what things can you do to ease this situation?

"Don't be ashamed of your story, it will inspire others!"

Day 6

How do I feel today? Circle the face that best represents how you feel.

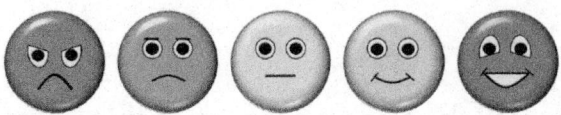

Record any observations and feelings you are experiencing, both positive and negative, in the space below.

Day 6

Day 6 - Bee kind to yourself!

Self -care. In sobriety everything is more real. You laugh more and it's hearty, and when you are sad – oh my gosh you will cry and you will feel it! When this happens and you're no longer a victim of the alcohol trap thinking that alcohol is self-care, you need to have alternatives. True self-care is about face masks, hot baths, meditation, exercise, and healing. Your mission is easy today! Run a hot bath and light a candle. Indulge! Then look in the mirror and appreciate how amazing you are!

Ideas:

- Go for a walk/exercise.
- Reward yourself.
- Plan something special.
- Take a hot bath.
- Affirm your worth.
- Meditate.
- Go offline for the day.
- Sing your favourite song loudly.
- Cook something special.
- Keep hydrated.
- Spend time reading.
- De-clutter your social media accounts.
- Try breathing exercises.
- Laugh.
- Go to bed early or sleep in late.

- Sit in the grass and watch the clouds float by.
- Do yoga.
- Do something crafty: colouring, knitting, sewing.
- Take a mental health day — and feel not an ounce of guilt about it.
- Watch the sun rise or set. Don't take any pictures or post about it on social media. Just watch.
- Say "no" to someone.

Day 6 Activity

Today, look after yourself. Spend the day doing things that make you feel good. Treat yourself to a nice bath, light a candle and tell yourself how gorgeous and amazing you are in the mirror!

"Life begins at the edge of your comfort zone"

Day 7

How do I feel today? Circle the face that best represents how you feel.

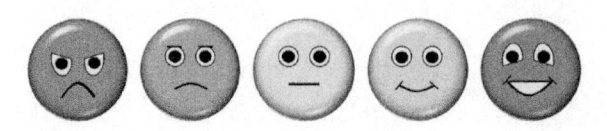

Record any observations and feelings you are experiencing, both positive and negative, in the space below.

Day 7

Day 7 - Anxiety

Anxiety. Anxiety seems to be a common trait amongst drinkers. Either they drink because they believe it relieves anxiety – to get a bit of "Dutch courage" or they suffer with "hangxiety" after drinking. What you will find is once you give up the booze, you need new healthy ways to manage your anxiety. You may become more aware of your anxiety after giving up the booze or you may find that it disappears altogether once you allow your brain chemistry to stabilise. Either way, an excellent way of managing anxiety is getting close to nature and feeling the moment. Take a walk, do it mindfully – really feel it!

Day 7 Activity

Walking is a great exercise and brilliant for relieving stress, Over the next week we suggest that you go for at least 1 X 15-30 minute walk each day. A great time to go would be when you would normally open a bottle of wine or beer.

Walking is a genius way to change habits, there is no need to go anywhere special all you need is an open mind. The aim is to go as mindfully as you can, focusing on your feet as they land on the ground, pay attention to all the sights, the trees swaying, birds flapping, etc. Every moment no matter what season, regardless of where you live has a host of sensory delights that will soon have you not only forgetting about drinking but feeling grateful that you aren't.

Week One Evaluation

Use this page to record how you are feeling at the end of each week.

What have you enjoyed most in the last week?

What has surprised you the most?

What is your top tip to yourself for next week?

What has been your biggest challenge this week and how did you overcome it?

"You can do it! You've got this!"

Day 8

How do I feel today? Circle the face that best represents how you feel.

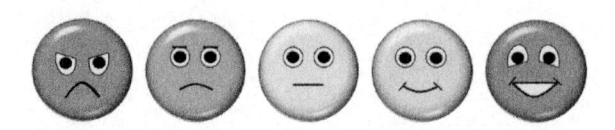

Record any observations and feelings you are experiencing, both positive and negative, in the space below.

Day 8

Day 8 - The Alcohol Industry

The Alcohol Industry. This is similar to what we did on day four but this time we want you to pay specific attention to the alcohol industry. The alcohol industry makes billions of pounds out of putting poison into drinks and disguising a taste that would not only repulse you in its neat form, but could even kill you if you had only a small amount. Today we want you to wake up. How does the alcohol industry cleverly make you crave a drink? Notice all the ways the dangers get overlooked! Come on, have you ever seen a drunk person advertising the very product they're selling? Nope! Vomiting, slurring and staggering just wouldn't cut it!

Day 8 Activity

When you are out and about, notice all the different ways that the alcohol industry works to persuade you to have a drink and how the dangers of alcohol are deliberately overlooked.

"You can be pitiful or powerful, you cannot be both"

Day 9

How do I feel today? Circle the face that best represents how you feel.

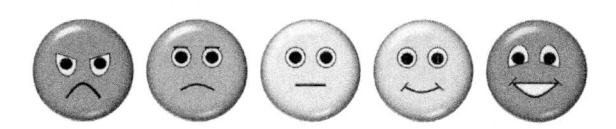

Record any observations and feelings you are experiencing, both positive and negative, in the space below.

Day 9

Day 9 - Positive Thinking

Positive thinking. Have you ever told yourself you can't have something? Have you then noticed you want it even more? Giving up alcohol requires more than gritting your teeth and going for it. Not only is it extremely addictive, making you crave it, but it is absolutely everywhere you look. This is why it is so important to change the way you think and feel about it and it begins with the way you think and feel about yourself. Once you start to realise your self-worth, you will no longer want to poison yourself. You are worth more. So, let's get started with a few affirmations – practice these daily, starting today.

Day 9 Activity

Write down three affirmations and recite them to yourself daily and throughout the day:

Examples:
I like myself
I am enough
I am worthy of living a life without alcohol

You can even take a photo of them and save them to your phone as a constant reminder of how amazing you are.

_____

_____

_____

"You are not a failure at drinking, you are a success at not drinking"

Day 10

How do I feel today? Circle the face that best represents how you feel.

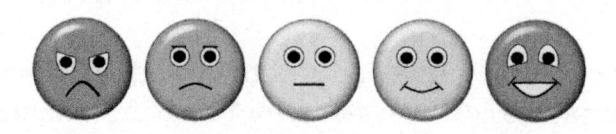

Record any observations and feelings you are experiencing, both positive and negative, in the space below.

Day 10

Day 10 – Meditation

Meditation. Practice meditating. Start small – just a couple of minutes each day has amazing health benefits and the beauty is, there's no right or wrong way to do this. Meditation has been scientifically proven to reduce stress, control anxiety, promote good emotional and mental health, enhance self-awareness, lengthen your attention span, improve memory (including age-related memory loss) and help with addiction.

Day 10 Activity

Spend one- or two-minutes practicing meditation. If this is something you feel could relax you or help you to focus, build it into your morning routine.

"The more comfortable you are with your negative emotions, the less you will resort to covering them up"

Day 11

How do I feel today? Circle the face that best represents how you feel.

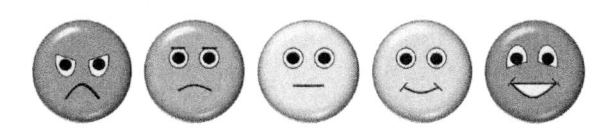

Record any observations and feelings you are experiencing, both positive and negative, in the space below.

Day 11

Day 11 – I Don't Drink

I don't drink! How do you stop people constantly trying to get you to have a drink? For some people, this can be a stumbling block. We want you to become sober and proud to be sober. It takes practice and an air of confidence to get this right. So today, stand facing a mirror. Loudly and proudly say "No thank you, I don't drink". This is where you want to get to, but for now, the main thing is what you tell yourself. That's right, it's more positive mindset work. Simply switching from "I can't drink" to "I choose not to drink" can be extremely empowering.

Day 11 Activity

Practice looking in the mirror and saying out loud "No thank you, I don't drink". Say it with assertiveness and with positivity. Own the phrase with confidence and know that this was your choice and not something to be pitied over. Take out "I can't" and replace with "I choose not to" in your tone.

"Make your sober story louder than your drinking story"

Day 12

How do I feel today? Circle the face that best represents how you feel.

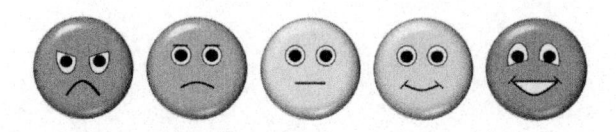

Record any observations and feelings you are experiencing, both positive and negative, in the space below.

Day 12

Day 12 – Social Life

Will I still have a social life? When you stop drinking, it can feel like you are giving up your social life. That doesn't have to be the case. For some people, going to the pub like you used to do can be too much and can be a huge trigger, so avoid it. For others, they manage to do this relatively easily (usually because they have nailed day 11). Whatever happens, no one should be locked away because they choose a better lifestyle. So, what else could you do? Get searching sober social groups or take up a new (or old) hobby with friends. Start small and you'll soon be a sober social butterfly!

Day 12 Activity

What activities will you do when socialising. Research sober social groups and/or find activities in your area that you would enjoy doing with family and friends. Write a list below.

"Don't judge or look at my past too hard, I don't live there anymore!"

Day 13

How do I feel today? Circle the face that best represents how you feel.

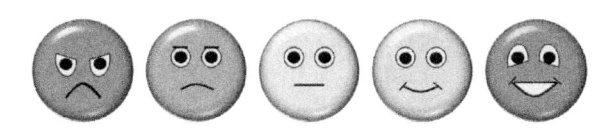

Record any observations and feelings you are experiencing, both positive and negative, in the space below.

Day 13

Day 13 – Mindset

Mindset. Have you met your wine witch yet? If so, you will already have heard the inner whisperings of temptation. Around day 13, it is so easy to feel you have managed it and can go back to moderation. In reality, moderation is rarely achievable, and when it is, it is blooming hard work. Today, we want you put the wine witch in her place. Remind yourself why you stopped drinking. Write your inner voice a letter and be honest.

Day 13 Activity

Write a letter to your inner voice. Tell it what you are doing about stopping drinking and why you are doing it. Write down how mean and cruel it is being to you and tell it your new beliefs. If you find this difficult, imagine writing it to a real person who has said these things to you or someone you love.

*"May you have the courage to
break the patterns in your life that
are no longer serving you"*

Day 14

How do I feel today? Circle the face that best represents how you feel.

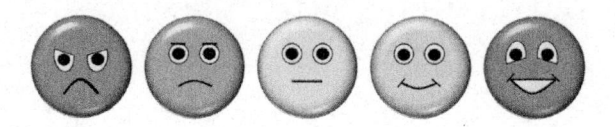

Record any observations and feelings you are experiencing, both positive and negative, in the space below.

Day 14

Day 14 – Sugar Cravings

Sugar cravings. Did you believe you would lose weight when you stopped drinking and have you found you haven't? Could it be the chocolate and cake that you now seem to eat so much of? Go easy on yourself. Alcoholic drinks are absolutely loaded with sugar so that you actually enjoy them. It's is no wonder that when you cut them out, you replace drinking with eating. Over time you can deal with this properly and the weight loss might happen. For now, at best, you should allow yourself the odd cake/chocolate bar and where possible, find healthier alternatives.

Day 14 Activity

Use the table to create a healthy alternative list for your sugary foods.

Sugary foods I eat	Alternative healthy foods

Week Two Evaluation

Use this page to record how you are feeling at the end of each week.

What have you enjoyed most in the last week?

What has surprised you the most?

What is your top tip to yourself for next week?

What has been your biggest challenge this week and how did you overcome it?

"You cannot always control what goes on outside, but you can control what goes on inside"

Day 15

How do I feel today? Circle the face that best represents how you feel.

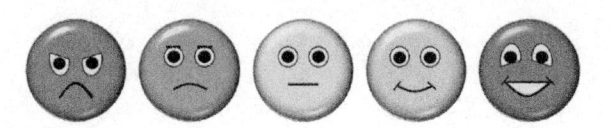

Record any observations and feelings you are experiencing, both positive and negative, in the space below.

Day 15

Day 15 – Moderation

Moderation. Have you tried moderating alcohol before? "Tonight, I will only drink three glasses, I won't drink in the week, I won't drink spirits". Moderation can mean different things to different people and depends on individual drinking habits. One thing it does have in common for everyone, is the effort it takes to maintain it. If you are someone who has tried and failed to moderate, as so many of us have, how can you be sure whether you're managing to moderate or not? In reality, the majority of people doing this experiment are doing it for the very reason that they haven't managed to moderate successfully. Learning what moderation means to you can be a good starting point.

Day 15 Activity

What does moderation look like to you? Write down exactly what this means in terms of which drinks are acceptable, how many, how often. At what point would you recognise you have drunk too much and not managed to moderate?

Time to Bee Honest - Alcohol myths and facts.

Misguided beliefs about drinking may fuel your choices or the choices of a loved one. Learning the facts may be helpful in making the best decisions regarding alcohol.

Myth: Alcohol helps me sleep?
Fact: Alcohol disrupts sleep cycles; it literally just knocks you out.

Myth: Alcohol helps me relax
Fact: Alcohol causes stimulants to be released into your bloodstream which increases anxiety.

What do/did you believe alcohol did for you?

Is this true? Free yourself today from these old, outdated myths – add your own below

Myth:

Fact:

Myth:

Fact:

Myth:

Fact:

"Vulnerability is where innovation and creativity begin"

Day 16

How do I feel today? Circle the face that best represents how you feel.

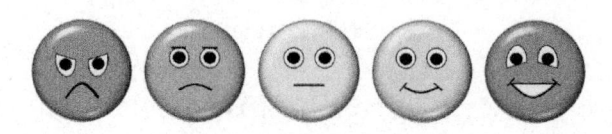

Record any observations and feelings you are experiencing, both positive and negative, in the space below.

Day 16

Day 16 – Mindfulness

Mindfulness. Have you ever truly thought about why you drink and what you actually enjoy about drinking? What triggers your cravings to drink? At what points are you perfectly content without a drink? How can you recognise and relieve triggers so that you don't pick up a drink today? Simply understanding the points in your day, or situations and circumstances that make you want to drink can help you to build new healthier habits instead of reaching for the booze.

Day 16 Activity

What are your triggers for drinking? What exactly will you do the next time you experience one?

"You are the one you have been waiting for"

Day 17

How do I feel today? Circle the face that best represents how you feel.

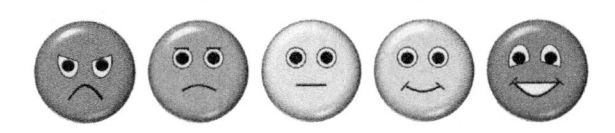

😠 😟 😐 🙂 😄

Record any observations and feelings you are experiencing, both positive and negative, in the space below.

Day 17

Day 17 – Won't Power

Won't power. How many times have you heard this: " wow, what amazing willpower to give up drinking"? Doesn't that just make you think how horrible stopping is going to be? How grueling and torturous it will be to use all your energy and strength to not reach for a drink today? We have big news for you! Quitting the alcohol doesn't have to be that way. You do not have to spend your life feeling as though you are missing out and lacking something in your life that you miss and crave. A shift in mindset to focus on all the reasons you don't want to drink alcohol, the truths around it and the risks associated with it can be one of the biggest tools in the sober toolbox and help you to actually not want it.

Day 17 Activity

Write down a list of alcohol truths. Find things that worry you about alcohol, for example, alcohol increases the risk of mouth cancer. When you next experience a craving, refer back to this list as a reminder.

"My choice not to drink is not a criticism of your choice to drink"

Day 18

How do I feel today? Circle the face that best represents how you feel.

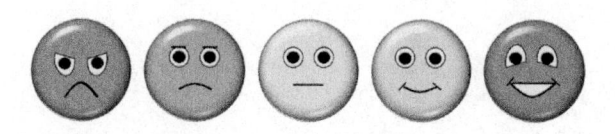

Record any observations and feelings you are experiencing, both positive and negative, in the space below.

Day 18

Day 18 – Boredom

Boredom. In the early days, even for people who didn't drink every day, time seems to expand in sobriety. Suddenly, you are waking earlier, you aren't mindlessly drinking your weekend away and time doesn't fly by in a blur. It is during this time you can start to crave alcohol as the boredom kicks in and you simply don't know what to do with yourself. You are an adult, yet you don't know what to do other than drink in your spare time. When was the last time you played a board game, went to the cinema, walked in the woods, did some exercise, meditated, played your guitar, danced like a crazy person or picked up an old hobby? Now is the time to find yourself all over again and achieve your life dreams. Sobriety is the gift that keeps on giving.

Day 18 Activity

What are your hopes and dreams? What have you always wanted to do but either told yourself you can't or haven't even attempted? Which one(s) are you willing to try?

"You have not failed until the day you stop trying"

Day 19

How do I feel today? Circle the face that best represents how you feel.

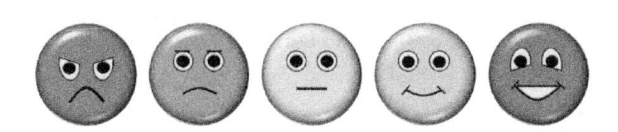

Record any observations and feelings you are experiencing, both positive and negative, in the space below.

Day 19

Day 19 – Stress

Stress. Many people drink to self-medicate their stressful lives. Whether that be a drink to "help" wind down at the end of the day or week, or a drink to take the edge of a stressful life event. Alcohol is actually a depressant and will NEVER help you deal with stress. Sure, it numbs the initial feelings and makes you feel temporarily more relaxed, but when you wake up the next morning, the stress that caused you to drink in the first place will still be there. Not only is the stress still there, you now have a hangover to deal with and as the body has tried to counter the effects of the alcohol by producing stimulants, often you haven't slept well and suffer from "hangxiety" or beer fear! Healthy stress busters can help and over time, with a clear head, you will learn how to tackle all life situations head-on!

Day 19 Activity

Nurture a plant
This is one of our favorites. With some of the money you have saved from not drinking this week, we suggest you go and treat yourself to a new plant.

Nurturing a plant can have surprisingly big benefits and all they need in order to live and grow are 4 basic elements: air, water, nutrients and sunlight.

Plants are known to reduce stress, and create a feeling of well-being, so why not treat yourself and at the same time brighten up your home or workplace.

"What if everything you are going through leads you to everything you asked for?"

Day 20

How do I feel today? Circle the face that best represents how you feel.

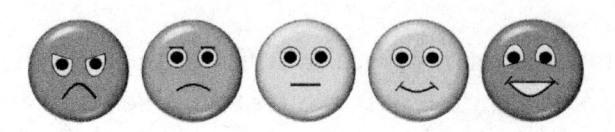

Record any observations and feelings you are experiencing, both positive and negative, in the space below.

Day 20

Day 20 – Meeting New People

Meeting new people. Quitting drinking can cause you to re-evaluate your social circle. If everyone you know drinks, it can be challenging. At some point, you need to make sober friends and what about sober dating? Many people use alcohol to give them a bit of Dutch courage, and without it, you can feel exposed and vulnerable. Taking a few well-planned steps to meet new people who just "get it", can help you to achieve a full and happy social life. Laughs will be louder; conversation will be deeper and memories will be made. You can start small with this one, joining a sober support group on Facebook, following sober accounts on Instagram or simply meeting up with existing friends for coffee or a walk, away from alcohol, can help you to gain confidence around sober socialising.

Day 20 Activity

Think about ways you can meet new people. List your dating ideas (or other socialising ideas). Make them fun and creative.

"Stop shrinking yourself into the places you no longer fit – you've simply outgrown them"

Day 21

How do I feel today? Circle the face that best represents how you feel.

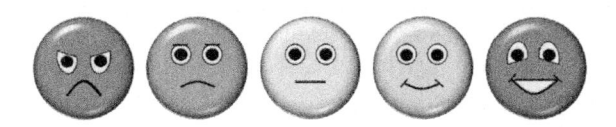

Record any observations and feelings you are experiencing, both positive and negative, in the space below.

Day 21

Day 21 – Effects on the body

Effects on the body. When we ask people what kills those who drink too much, they usually answer Liver disease. And whilst that is true, it is not the biggest killer. Stroke and Heart Attack are the biggest killers. Did you also know alcohol causes seven different types of cancer? Bowel, breast, laryngeal, liver, mouth, oesophageal and pharyngeal. As humans we always think it will happen to someone else and we won't be that statistic. Often, even knowing the risks won't stop us. However, it can help to serve as a useful reminder that alcohol is a poison that we are literally soaking our organs in. Did you know it was banned for use as an anaesthetic in the 1970s because it was too toxic? Speaking of anaesthesia, if you do drink alcohol before surgery, you are at a significantly higher risk of death or complications!

Day 21 Activity

Take a photo of yourself or draw a head-to-toe self-portrait (it doesn't have to be a masterpiece, but it does have to represent you) and glue it or draw it in the space below. Label all the parts of the body that alcohol could damage if you continued to drink as you previously did.

Week Three Evaluation

Use this page to record how you are feeling at the end of each week.

What have you enjoyed most in the last week?

What has surprised you the most?

What is your top tip to yourself for next week?

What has been your biggest challenge this week and how did you overcome it?

"I am not what I have done, I am what I have overcome"

Day 22

How do I feel today? Circle the face that best represents how you feel.

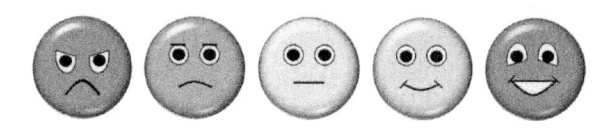

Record any observations and feelings you are experiencing, both positive and negative, in the space below.

Day 22

Day 22 – Power of the Mind

Power of the mind. Your mind can be your most powerful enemy or your most powerful ally! Have you ever had a bad day and everything just seems to go wrong? Most of that is honestly down to mindset. A simple switch, a fake smile, a bit of loud dance music and things can turn around quite dramatically. Knowing this can mean you can use your mind as a tool. When you next have a social occasion or situation where you might encounter alcohol, visualise how you want it to be. Think about what you will wear, what you will order at the bar, visualise dancing and chatting or relaxing with your favourite person. Write down your vision of how the event will be and compare it to the reality – you might just surprise yourself!

Day 22 Activity

When is your next social occasion? Visualise how you want it to be. Visualise all the fun elements, even the things you believe drink helped you with. This might be dancing, chatting to strangers or just relaxing with one person who you are ease with. Write down (or record a video/voice note) a description of this visualisation. After the occasion, record what actually happened.

My Visualisation:

Record of my Event:

"Let go of who you think you are supposed to be and embrace who you are" Brené Brown

Day 23

How do I feel today? Circle the face that best represents how you feel.

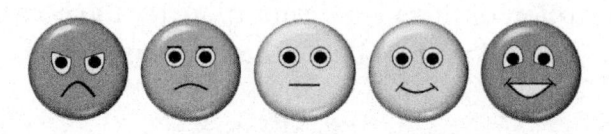

Record any observations and feelings you are experiencing, both positive and negative, in the space below.

Day 23

Day 23 – Advertising

Advertising. So, we have already looked at the ways that alcohol has been sold to you over the years and if you're anything like us, it'll make you a bit angry that you have been tricked. When you start to realise that the very product of drinking (a drunk person) is never used to advertise alcohol, surely you have to think about why. Do you honestly think alcohol would sell if the adverts showed vomiting, fighting, blacking out, weeing in the street, cheating on partners and other hideous yet "normal" drunken incidences? How should alcohol be advertised. What would an honest advert to your younger self look like now your eyes are wide open?

Day 23 Activity

Write an advertisement to your younger self about why you shouldn't start drinking.

"The expert in anything was also once a beginner"

Day 24

How do I feel today? Circle the face that best represents how you feel.

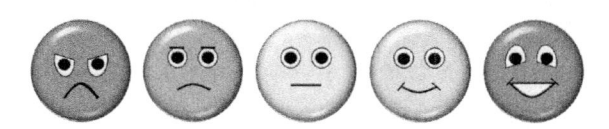

Record any observations and feelings you are experiencing, both positive and negative, in the space below.

Day 24

Day 24 – Feeling Angry

Feeling angry. When was the last time you got angry? What happened to trigger it? What did you do? Often, anger comes from somewhere else. It arises from fear, stress, frustration or anxiety about a situation or circumstance. There is a really good reason for counting to 10 when you feel angry, it allows you to process the root cause and often just nips it in the bud. Anger is, however, a perfectly normal human emotion, so give yourself a break. Next time you feel angry, try to look beneath it. What is really going on? Now practice techniques for dealing with is, scream into a pillow, exercise vigorously, shake it out!

Day 24 Activity

Look beneath you last anger episode. What was the real feeling beneath the anger? What was the cause?

"Everyone you meet is fighting a battle you know nothing about. Be kind."

Day 25

How do I feel today? Circle the face that best represents how you feel.

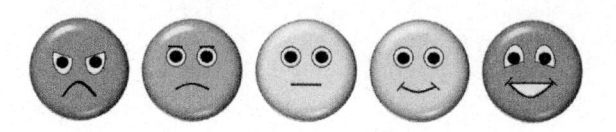

Record any observations and feelings you are experiencing, both positive and negative, in the space below.

Day 25

Day 25 – Depression

Depression. Alcohol only adds to or causes depression. That is because, alcohol is a depressant drug. It does not have the ability to make you feel good over the long term, so if you are someone who suffers from depression or even sadness, alcohol will exacerbate it. People sometimes use alcohol to self-medicate or numb their sadness but it never takes away the root cause. Using alcohol means you never actually deal with the cause of the depression and many people remain undiagnosed because they didn't even know they were suffering depression. So many sober people seek therapy in their sobriety when they realise there are events or trauma that they didn't address and you may also decide to do that. In the meantime, there are simple things that you can do to start feeling more positive. Start by thinking what (other than drugs or alcohol) truly makes you feel happy? Why not try to do more of it with all this extra time you seem to have now?

Day 25 Activity

Identify one thing (not alcohol or drugs) that makes you truly happy (or used to make you truly happy) when you are doing it. Build it in to your week this week.

*"You've got a new story to write
and it looks nothing like your past"*

Day 26

How do I feel today? Circle the face that best represents how you feel.

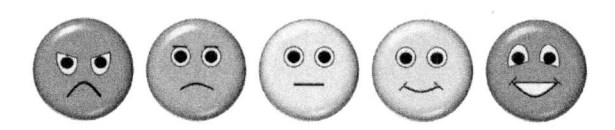

Record any observations and feelings you are experiencing, both positive and negative, in the space below.

Day 26

Day 26 – Effects on ageing

Effects of ageing. It's selfie day. Get that day two selfie out and compare. With three weeks sobriety under your belt, you will be seeing and/or feeling the differences. Have the shadows under your eyes started to fade? What about dry skin, blemishes and wrinkles? What do your hair and nails look and feel like? What physical differences can you see and feel? Alcohol ages you and your brain, not least because it is a toxin that you are pouring into your body and soaking into your cells. Even at this stage, the lack of dehydration will start to show. Let us know your thoughts on this one and if you're brave enough, post those selfies in the group.

Day 26 Activity

Take another selfie. If you can, print the one from day 2 and the one from today and stick them below. Record your observations. If you cannot print them, create a before and after picture on your phone (or send it to us soberexperiment@gmail.com) and we will do it for you.

"Push yourself, no one else will do this for you"

Day 27

How do I feel today? Circle the face that best represents how you feel.

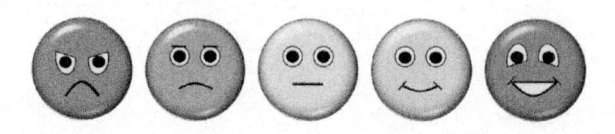

Record any observations and feelings you are experiencing, both positive and negative, in the space below.

Day 27

Day 27 – Benefits

Benefits. When that voice starts chatting in your head, what does it say to you? Does it say things you wouldn't say to your worst enemy? Write down negative things you say to yourself or about yourself to others. Now reframe them. For example, you could change "I haven't lost any weight during sobriety, what's the point?" into "I feel amazing and this will soon start to show in my weight if I keep going", or how about "I hate being the only sober one at the party, I am so boring" into "I choose to be sober, I don't end up talking shit to everyone and am always so grateful in the morning when I am the only one without a hangover". Mindset is very powerful in sobriety – give this a try.

Day 27 Activity

Observe your language. Write down three negative things you either say to yourself or say to others about yourself (especially if they are about you stopping drinking). Re-write these into positives.

"In a world full of chaos, ground yourself with the beautiful things going on in your life"

Day 28

How do I feel today? Circle the face that best represents how you feel.

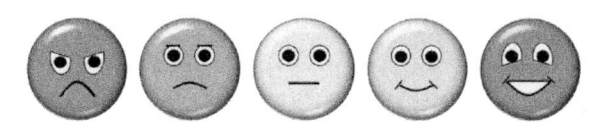

Record any observations and feelings you are experiencing, both positive and negative, in the space below.

Day 28

Day 28 – Gratitude

Gratitude. Referring to your day one activity can be really useful at this point. Why did you decide to try sober? What were your positives of not drinking and drinking? Over the last four weeks, what have you been truly grateful for that you wouldn't have experienced if you hadn't been sober? Being grateful, even for small things, even when things are not going well, can lead to fulfillment and greater happiness. Gratitude can also stop you feeling negative emotions such as resentment, envy or fear of missing out. A healthy mind often means a healthy body, practice gratitude – there's ALWAYS something to be grateful for.

What are the Benefits of Gratitude?

- increased happiness and positive mood
- more satisfaction with life
- less materialistic
- less likely to experience burnout
- better physical health
- better sleep
- less fatigue
- lower levels of cellular inflammation
- greater resiliency
- encourages the development of patience, humility, and wisdom

Day 28 Activity

We now want you to start concentrating on all the things you are grateful for. Gratitude has huge benefits and is strongly and consistently associated with greater happiness.

Gratitude also helps magnify your positive emotions and helps block negative emotions like envy, resentment and regret meaning it will help you feel more positivity, relish good experiences, improve health, deal with adversity and build strong relationships.

So, today we would like you to list at least 10 things you are grateful for:

"What you allow is what will continue"

Day 29

How do I feel today? Circle the face that best represents how you feel.

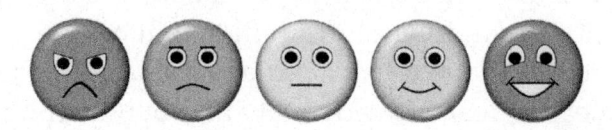

Record any observations and feelings you are experiencing, both positive and negative, in the space below.

Day 29

Day 29 – Taking Control

Taking control. During the last few weeks, you will have faced cravings, triggers, stress, anxiety, worry and many more negative emotions and experiences. If you have got to this point sober, you have clearly built a toolbox that has allowed you to be resilient. You didn't crack! If you did relapse at any point, you will have learnt lessons. What made you relapse and what would you do next time that situation arises? These are the tools that you are building in your sober toolbox that you have been hearing from everyone in the sober sphere. There is no right or wrong in this toolbox, it is very personal to you and you will keep building it. So, what is in it?

Day 29 Activity

What tools do you have in your 'sober toolbox'? IF you relapsed, what could you do to get you back on track?

Week Four Evaluation

Use this page to record how you are feeling at the end of each week.

What have you enjoyed most in the last week?

What has surprised you the most?

What is your top tip to yourself for next week?

What has been your biggest challenge this week and how did you overcome it?

"Be stronger than your excuses"

Day 30

How do I feel today? Circle the face that best represents how you feel.

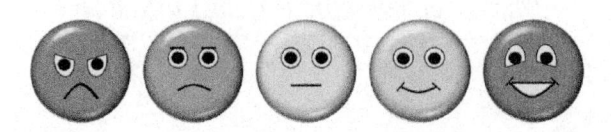

Record any observations and feelings you are experiencing, both positive and negative, in the space below.

Day 30

Day 30 – Your Decision

Your decision. So, we are at the end of the experiment. Or are we? What will it be? Will you carry on for a bit longer, go back to the alcohol or quit for good? Will you try to moderate? Whatever your decision, it is yours and yours alone. We are not magicians and we never promised this journey would be easy, but we did promise it would be worth it. If you decide to moderate, please ask yourself if the effort will be worth it. If you were a successful moderator then why did you want to take a break? If you decide to go back to drinking as you did before, go back to your WHY. Why did you take a break? If you decide this is forever, great – it gets better and better and better. And if you decide to try for a little bit longer, keep in touch via DM so we can support you along the way. Whatever you decide, we are glad you gave this a go and gave yourself the gift of sobriety. You smashed it!

Day 30 Activity

What are your current pros of drinking alcohol and not drinking alcohol? Now compare these to day one. What are the similarities and differences? Use this to inform your decision about what you do next!

Pros of drinking alcohol	Pros of not drinking alcohol

Useful Numbers

Alcoholics Anonymous - Great Britain

AA is an organisation of men and women who share their experience with each other hoping to solve their problems and help others to recover from alcoholism. If you need help with a drinking problem, you can contact Alcoholics Anonymous.
Free helpline: 0800 917 7650
Email helpline: help@aamail.org

Al-Anon

Al-Anon is worldwide and offers support and understanding to the families and friends of problem drinkers.
Confidential Helpline 0800 008 6811 (open 10am-10pm)

Bee Sober CIC

Providing a supportive community to get and stay Sober
Email: info@beesoberofficial.com
Website: www.beesoberofficial.com

Drinkline

Drinkline runs a free, confidential helpline for people who are concerned about their drinking, or someone else's, regardless of the callers age, gender, sexuality, ethnicity or spirituality.
Free helpline: 0300 123 1110 (weekdays 9am–8pm, weekends 11am–4pm)

Hub of hope

The hub of hope is completely anonymous and basically a database that allows anyone, anywhere to find the nearest source of support for any mental health issue, from depression and anxiety to PTSD and suicidal thoughts it has a 'talk now' button too which connects you directly to the Samaritans.
You can download the Hub of Hope app by searching on your app store or click on the link below to find help near you.
https://hubofhope.co.uk/

Livewell by NHS Choices

Numerous easy-to-read resources on a variety of addictions, how to get help and self-service questionnaires. Available at
https://www.nhs.uk/Livewell/Addiction/Pages/addictionhome.aspx

National Association for Children of Alcoholics (NACOA)

Information, advice and support to children of alcohol-dependent parents and people concerned with their welfare through a free and confidential telephone and email helpline.
Free helpline: 0800 358 3456
Email helpline: helpline@nacoa.org.uk

National Domestic Abuse Helpline

0808 2000 247

Public Health England

A list of resources, reading material and treatment information for users, families, carers and healthcare professionals. Available at http://www.nta.nhs.uk/

Rehab Online

A directory of residential rehabilitation services across the UK. Users can search by location or by need. Available at http://www.rehab-online.org.uk/

Samaritans

Provides confidential non-judgmental emotional support, 24 hours a day for people who are experiencing feelings of distress, despair or suicide.
Helpline: 116 123 (24hrs)
Email helpline: jo@samaritans.org (they try their hardest to get back to your email within 24 hours)

Supportline

Confidential emotional support for rape and sexual assault survivors
Helpline: 01708 765200
Email: info@supportline.org.uk

Thank you for participating in The Sober Experiment® by Bee Sober.

This member's pack has armed you with the tools to make informed choices about your alcohol consumption. You now have the choice to return to your old ways, moderate your drinking using mindful drinking, or stay sober for longer. This is your decision and yours alone.

Whatever you choose, we hope you have found this useful and that you agree that taking part has changed your relationship with alcohol. We wish you the best of luck in the future, whatever you decide. Please take a minute to write us a short review and email it to us:

info@beesoberofficial.com

By purchasing this member's pack, you are helping to raise money for our non-profit organisation. Your money helps us to fund the podcast and allows us to continue to support the community.

Find out more www.beesoberofficial.com

Printed in Great Britain
by Amazon